ILEOSTOMY DIET COOKBOOK

A Guide to Delicious and Nutritious Meals After Ileostomy Surgery

SELENA LEONARD

Copyright© 2023 [Selena Leonard]

Table of Contents

Introduction

Embark on a Delicious Journey of Healing and Well-Being After Ileostomy Surgery

Following ileostomy surgery, navigating the world of food can feel overwhelming. The uncertainty of what to eat and the fear of complications can leave you feeling restricted and isolated. But what if you could reclaim the joy of eating and discover a world of delicious, nutritious meals specifically designed to support your healing and well-being?

This comprehensive cookbook, Ileostomy Diet Cookbook: A Guide to Delicious and Nutritious Meals After Ileostomy Surgery, is your empowering companion on this new chapter of your life. We understand the unique dietary needs following ileostomy surgery, and we're here to guide you every step of the way.

Within these pages, you'll find:

- Clear explanations of the impact of ileostomy surgery on digestion and absorption of nutrients.

- Essential information on the importance of proper nutrition for optimal healing and long-term health.

- A wealth of delicious and easy-to-follow recipes, carefully crafted using ileostomy-friendly ingredients.

- Practical tips and strategies for managing common digestive concerns after surgery.

- Empowering guidance on maintaining hydration and overall well-being.

This is not just a cookbook; it's a roadmap to rediscovering the pleasure of food and reclaiming control over your health. With our simple and flavorful recipes, you'll not only nourish your body but also rediscover the joy of cooking and sharing meals with loved ones.

So, join us on this culinary adventure, and embark on a journey of delicious healing and vibrant well-being after ileostomy surgery. Let's explore a world of flavor and possibility, together.

Part 1: Ileostomy Diet Essentials

Chapter 1:

Navigating the Early Days: Post-Surgery Diet Guidelines

Understanding the Immediate Post-Surgery Diet:

The first few days after ileostomy surgery are crucial for healing and establishing a new digestive rhythm. During this initial period, your healthcare team will likely recommend a clear liquid diet, followed by a gradual introduction of solid foods.

Recommended Foods and Fluids:

These clear liquids provide essential hydration and minimal digestive burden:

- ✓ Water: Your primary source of hydration. Aim for 8-10 glasses daily.
- ✓ Clear broths: Chicken, vegetable, or beef broth.
- ✓ Electrolyte beverages: Help replenish electrolytes lost through fluids. Choose low-sugar options.
- ✓ Apple juice: Diluted with water for better tolerance.

✓ Clear gelatin: Plain or flavored.

Gradually Introducing Solid Foods:

Once your healthcare team approves, you can begin incorporating solid foods, starting with easily digestible options. Here are some recommended foods:

- ✓ Well-cooked, lean meats: Chicken, turkey, fish (flaked or well-mashed).
- ✓ Starchy vegetables: Cooked potatoes, carrots, sweet potatoes, peas.
- ✓ Canned fruits: Peaches, pears, apricots (in small amounts and well-peeled).
- ✓ Well-cooked eggs: Scrambled or soft-boiled.
- ✓ White bread and crackers: Toast, bagels, crackers.
- ✓ Yogurt: Plain or flavored yogurt, but monitor lactose tolerance.
- ✓ Smoothies: Made with yogurt, banana, and cooked oats (blended smooth to avoid fiber).

Foods to Avoid or Limit:

Certain foods can irritate the digestive system or pose a risk of blockage, especially during the early recovery stages. It's best to avoid or limit these until your healthcare team advises otherwise:

- ✓ High-fiber foods: Raw fruits and vegetables, whole grains, nuts, seeds, and popcorn.
- ✓ Spicy foods: Can irritate the digestive system.
- ✓ Fatty foods: Fried foods, greasy meats, and processed foods can be difficult to digest.
- ✓ Dairy products: Monitor your tolerance for lactose. Some individuals may experience gas or bloating.
- ✓ Carbonated beverages: Can cause gas and bloating.
- ✓ Alcohol: Consult your healthcare team for guidance on alcohol consumption.
- ✓ Foods known to cause blockages: Grape skins, popcorn, certain meats (not chewed well), potato skins, mushrooms, pineapple, asparagus spears, tomato skins.

Managing Hydration:

Maintaining proper hydration is crucial throughout your entire recovery journey. Aim for 8-10 glasses of water daily, and consider additional options like:

- ✓ Electrolyte beverages: Replenish lost electrolytes, especially during hot weather or physical activity.
- ✓ Clear broths: Count towards your fluid intake and provide additional electrolytes.
- ✓ Herbal teas: Choose soothing options like chamomile or peppermint.
- ✓ Infused water: Add fruits, herbs, or cucumbers to water for a refreshing twist.

Recipe Example:

Creamy Banana Oatmeal Smoothie:

This smoothie provides essential nutrients and is gentle on the digestive system.

Ingredients:

- 1/2 banana

- 1/4 cup cooked oats

- 1/4 cup plain yogurt

- 1/2 cup unsweetened almond milk

- 1/4 teaspoon ground cinnamon (optional)

Instructions:

- Blend all ingredients together until smooth and creamy.

- Enjoy chilled.

Chapter 2:

Essential Nutrients for Optimal Health

Following ileostomy surgery, your body requires a balanced and varied diet to promote optimal healing, maintain energy levels, and prevent nutrient deficiencies. This chapter delves into the essential nutrients your body needs and how to incorporate them into your ileostomy diet.

Understanding Macronutrients and Micronutrients:

Nutrients can be broadly categorized into two groups:

Macronutrients: These are required in larger amounts and provide your body with energy. They include:

➤ Carbohydrates: Provide readily available energy. Choose complex carbohydrates like whole grains (once tolerated) and starchy vegetables over simple carbohydrates found in sugary drinks and processed foods.

➤ Proteins: Essential for building and repairing tissues, supporting immune function, and promoting satiety. Choose lean protein sources like chicken, fish, eggs, and legumes (once tolerated).

➤ Fats: Play a vital role in hormone production, cell function, and nutrient absorption. Opt for healthy fats found in avocados, nuts, seeds, and olive oil.

Micronutrients: These are needed in smaller quantities but are critical for various bodily functions, including:

➤ Vitamins: Essential for various metabolic processes, immunity, and overall health. Choose fruits and vegetables rich in vitamins A, C, D, E, and B complex.

➤ Minerals: Play crucial roles in bone health, muscle function, and nerve signaling. Include foods rich in calcium, potassium, iron, and magnesium in your diet.

Importance of Protein, Carbohydrates, Fats, Vitamins, and Minerals:

Each nutrient plays a specific and vital role in supporting your health after ileostomy surgery:

- ➤ Protein: Helps repair tissues, build muscle, and maintain a healthy immune system.
- ➤ Carbohydrates: Provide readily available energy for daily activities and healing.
- ➤ Fats: Aid in nutrient absorption, support cell health, and promote satiety.
- ➤ Vitamins: Ensure proper metabolic function, immune function, and overall well-being.
- ➤ Minerals: Contribute to strong bones, healthy muscles, and proper nerve function.

Choosing Nutrient-Rich Foods:

While navigating food restrictions after ileostomy surgery, it's crucial to prioritize nutrient-rich options. Here are some tips:

➢ Focus on variety: Include a diverse range of colors on your plate to ensure a broader spectrum of essential nutrients.

➢ Read food labels: Pay attention to nutrient content, choosing foods rich in protein, vitamins, and minerals while limiting added sugars, sodium, and unhealthy fats.

➢ Plan your meals: Planning helps ensure you incorporate all essential nutrients throughout the day.

➢ Consult a registered dietitian: They can provide personalized guidance on incorporating nutrient-rich options into your ileostomy-friendly diet.

➢ Examples of Nutrient-Rich Foods for an Ileostomy Diet:

➢ Protein: Skinless chicken or fish, eggs, tofu (once tolerated), lentils (once tolerated).

➤ Carbohydrates: White bread, crackers, cooked potatoes, sweet potatoes, bananas, applesauce.

➤ Fats: Avocados, nuts (ground or nut butter), olive oil.

➤ Vitamins: Leafy green vegetables, carrots, oranges, melons.

Minerals: Yogurt, fortified milk (once tolerated), bananas, potatoes.

Part 2: Meal Planning and Preparation

Chapter 3:

Stocking Your Pantry and Fridge: Ileostomy-Friendly Staples

Following ileostomy surgery, navigating the grocery store can feel overwhelming. This chapter equips you with the knowledge to stock your pantry and fridge with essential, ileostomy-friendly staples for delicious and nutritious meals at any time.

Essential Ingredients for Breakfast:

- Protein sources: Cooked chicken or turkey breast, canned tuna, eggs, low-fat Greek yogurt (once tolerated).
- Carbohydrates: White bread, bagels, crackers, cooked oats, bananas, applesauce.
- Healthy fats: Avocados, nut butters (smooth and no added sugar), olive oil.

> Other: Unsweetened almond milk, honey (limited), cinnamon, ground ginger.

Breakfast Recipe Example:

Scrambled Eggs with Toast and Avocado:

- Scramble 2 eggs with a splash of milk.
- Toast a slice of white bread.
- Mash 1/4 avocado and spread on the toast.
- Season with salt and pepper to taste.

Essential Ingredients for Lunch and Dinner:

> Protein sources: Skinless chicken or fish fillets, lean ground meat (once tolerated), canned beans/lentils (rinsed and drained, once tolerated), tofu (once tolerated).

> Vegetables: canned or frozen vegetables (cooked and well-mashed), cooked carrots, sweet potatoes, peas, and green beans.

➢ Starchy options: white rice, pasta, potatoes (mashed or baked).

➢ Healthy fats: olive oil, avocado oil, and nut butters.

➢ Seasonings: Herbs and spices like dried basil, oregano, garlic powder, onion powder, salt, and pepper.

Lunch & Dinner Recipe Example:

Baked Chicken Breast with Roasted Vegetables:

- Preheat oven to 400°F (200°C).

- Season boneless, skinless chicken breast with herbs and spices.

- Chop carrots, potatoes, and green beans.

- Toss vegetables with olive oil and spread on a baking sheet.

- Place chicken breast on top of the vegetables.

- Bake for 20–25 minutes, or until chicken is cooked through and vegetables are tender.

Essential Ingredients for Snacks:

- Fruits: bananas, applesauce, canned fruits (in moderation), melons (peeled and seeded).

- Protein sources: Smooth peanut butter, low-fat cheese, yogurt (once tolerated).

- Carbohydrates: Rice cakes, pretzels, crackers.

- Healthy fats: Avocados, nut butters.

Snack Recipe Example:

- Rice Cake with Peanut Butter and Banana:

- Spread smooth peanut butter on a rice cake.

- Top with sliced banana.

- Tips for Smart Shopping and Food Storage:

- Plan your meals: Create a weekly meal plan to avoid impulse purchases and ensure you have the necessary ingredients on hand.

- Buy in bulk: Purchase staples like rice, pasta, and canned goods in bulk when on sale, if storage space allows.

- Check expiration dates: Always check expiration dates before buying and prioritize items with longer shelf lives.

- Focus on fresh produce: Choose fresh fruits and vegetables in season for optimal taste and nutrient content.

- Proper storage: Store fruits and vegetables in the crisper drawer. Freeze fruits and vegetables for longer storage (if not planning to use them immediately). Store cooked foods in airtight containers in the refrigerator for up to 3 days.

- Portion control: Purchase pre-portioned single-serving snacks to avoid overeating.

By stocking your pantry and fridge with these ileostomy-friendly staples, you'll be well-equipped to prepare delicious and nutritious meals throughout the day. Remember, this list is a starting point, and individual tolerances may vary. Always follow the specific recommendations of your healthcare team and introduce new foods gradually, monitoring how your body reacts.

Chapter 4:

Meal Planning Tips for a Balanced and Varied Diet

After ileostomy surgery, navigating meal planning can seem challenging. However, with careful planning and organization, you can create delicious and nutritious meals that support your healing and well-being. This chapter equips you with essential tips for crafting balanced and varied meal plans that cater to your individual needs and preferences.

Creating Weekly Meal Plans:

➤ Start with your schedule: Consider your daily activities and allocate realistic meal and snack times.

➤ Set achievable goals: Aim for a variety of food groups at each meal, focusing on incorporating protein, carbohydrates, healthy fats, and essential vitamins and minerals.

➢ Involve loved ones: Include family or friends in the planning process for added support and motivation.

➢ Utilize online resources: Numerous websites and apps offer ileostomy-friendly recipes and meal planning tools.

➢ Balancing Meal Portions and Macronutrients:

➢ Portion control is key: Use measuring cups and spoons to ensure you're consuming appropriate serving sizes.

➢ The MyPlate method: This visual guide from the USDA provides a framework for balanced meals, encouraging half your plate to be filled with fruits and vegetables, a quarter with protein, and a quarter with grains.

Understanding macronutrients:

➢ Protein: Aim for 2 - 3 servings (3-4 ounces each) per day.

➢ Carbohydrates: Choose complex carbohydrates like whole grains (once tolerated) and starchy vegetables in moderation.

➤ Fats: Include healthy fats from sources like avocados, nuts, seeds, and olive oil.

Sample Meal Plan 1:

- Breakfast: Scrambled eggs with whole-wheat toast (if tolerated) and avocado.
- Lunch: Tuna salad sandwich on white bread with lettuce and tomato, side of canned peaches.
- Dinner: Baked chicken breast with roasted vegetables (carrots, sweet potatoes, green beans) and mashed potatoes.
- Snacks: Yogurt with berries, banana with peanut butter, rice cakes with cheese.

Sample Meal Plan 2:

- Breakfast: Smoothies made with banana, yogurt, and cooked oats (blended smooth).
- Lunch: Chicken noodle soup (made with broth, cooked chicken, carrots, and noodles) and crackers.

- Dinner: Baked fish with steamed broccoli and brown rice (if tolerated).

- Snacks: Applesauce, pretzels with nut butter, yogurt with chia seeds.

Remember: These are just sample meal plans, and individual needs and tolerances may vary. It is crucial to consult with your healthcare team for personalized dietary recommendations and portion sizes. They can also guide you on introducing new foods gradually and monitor your progress.

Additional Tips:

- Rotate proteins and vegetables: This ensures a variety of nutrients and keeps your meals interesting.

- Season your food with herbs and spices: This adds flavor without adding unnecessary salt or sugar.

- Don't be afraid to experiment: Try new recipes and find healthy options you enjoy.

- Stay hydrated: Drink plenty of water throughout the day to support digestion and overall well-being.

By incorporating these tips and working with your healthcare team, you can create sustainable and enjoyable meal plans that support your healing journey and promote long-term health after ileostomy surgery.

Part 3: Delicious and Easy Recipes

Chapter 5:

Breakfast Recipes: Fueling Your Day the Right Way

Kickstart your day with delicious and nutritious breakfasts that provide your body with the essential nutrients it needs for optimal healing and energy. This chapter features several easy-to-follow recipes specifically designed for an ileostomy diet, complete with nutritional information, instructions, and helpful tips.

Recipes

Creamy Banana Oatmeal Smoothie

(approx. 300 calories, 18g protein, 38g carbohydrates, 4g fat)

This smoothie provides a creamy and refreshing start to your day, packed with protein, carbohydrates, and fiber (from cooked oats).

Ingredients:

- 1/2 banana (peeled and frozen)

- 1/4 cup cooked oats (blended smooth)

- 1/4 cup plain yogurt (unsweetened or low-sugar)

- 1/2 cup unsweetened almond milk

- 1/4 teaspoon ground cinnamon (optional)

Instructions:

- Blend all ingredients together until smooth and creamy.

- Enjoy chilled.

Tips:

- Replace frozen banana with other frozen fruits like berries or mangoes for a variety of flavors.

- Add a scoop of protein powder for an extra protein boost.

- Use unsweetened plant-based milk for a dairy-free option.

Scrambled Eggs with Vegetables and Toast

(approx. 250 calories, 18g protein, 18g carbohydrates, 10g fat)

This classic breakfast is a great source of protein and healthy fats, featuring easy-to-digest scrambled eggs with colorful vegetables on toast.

Ingredients:

- 2 eggs
- 1 tablespoon milk (low-fat or unsweetened plant-based)
- 1/4 cup chopped vegetables (e.g., bell peppers, spinach, mushrooms)
- 1 slice white bread (toasted)
- Salt and pepper to taste
- Cooking spray

Instructions:

- Preheat a non-stick pan coated with cooking spray over medium heat.

- Whisk together eggs and milk in a bowl.

- Add vegetables to the pan and cook until softened, about 2-3 minutes.

- Pour in the egg mixture and scramble gently until cooked through.

- Season with salt and pepper to taste.

- Serve scrambled eggs on the toasted bread.

Tips:

- Use pre-chopped frozen vegetables for added convenience.

- Choose low-fiber vegetables like spinach or zucchini for easier digestion.

- Substitute sliced avocado for toast for a healthy fat and fiber boost (once tolerated).

Yogurt Parfait with Fruit and Granola

(modified) (approx. 200 calories, 8g protein, 30g carbohydrates, 3g fat)

This layered parfait offers a delightful combination of creamy yogurt, sweetness from fruit, and a satisfying crunch from crushed granola.

Ingredients:

- 1/2 cup plain yogurt (unsweetened or low-sugar)
- 1/4 cup sliced banana or other soft fruits (e.g., berries, melon)
- 2 tablespoons crushed granola (modified by coarsely grinding or using a commercially available soft granola option)

Instructions:

- Layer yogurt, fruit, and crushed granola in a small bowl or glass.
- Enjoy chilled.

Tips:

- Choose yogurt options labeled lactose-free if you have lactose intolerance.

- Crush granola in a mortar and pestle or food processor to avoid large pieces, which might be difficult to digest.

- Substitute crushed nuts or seeds for granola for extra protein and healthy fats (once tolerated).

Protein Pancakes

(approx. 250 calories, 20g protein, 25g carbohydrates, 5g fat):

Ingredients:

- 1/2 cup cooked oatmeal
- 1 scoop protein powder (unflavored or vanilla)
- 1/4 cup unsweetened almond milk
- 1 egg
- 1/4 teaspoon baking powder
- Optional: 1/4 teaspoon cinnamon

Instructions:

- Blend all ingredients until smooth.
- Preheat a lightly greased non-stick pan over medium heat.
- Pour 1/4 cup of batter per pancake.

- Cook for 2-3 minutes per side, or until golden brown and cooked through.
- Serve with a dollop of low-fat yogurt and fresh berries.

Tips:

- Use different protein powder flavors for variety.
- Add a pinch of stevia or a teaspoon of mashed banana for natural sweetness.
- Top with chopped nuts or seeds for added protein and healthy fats (once tolerated).

Baked Apples with Chia Seeds and Nuts

(approx. 200 calories, 4g protein, 40g carbohydrates, 5g fat):

Ingredients:

- 2 medium apples (cored)
- 1/4 cup sliced almonds
- 1 tablespoon chia seeds
- 1/4 teaspoon ground cinnamon

- 1 tablespoon unsweetened applesauce

Instructions:

- Preheat oven to 375°F (190°C).

- In a small bowl, combine sliced almonds, chia seeds, and cinnamon.

- Stuff the apple cores with the mixture.

- Top each apple with a dollop of applesauce.

- Bake for 20-25 minutes, or until apples are tender.

Tips:

- Use different types of nuts or seeds like chopped walnuts or pecans for a variety of flavors (once tolerated).

- Drizzle with a teaspoon of honey for a touch of sweetness (once tolerated).

- Substitute apples with pears for a different fruit option.

Cottage Cheese Bowl with Berries and Granola

(approx. 200 calories, 15g protein, 20g carbohydrates, 5g fat):

Ingredients:

- 1/2 cup low-fat cottage cheese
- 1/4 cup mixed berries
- 2 tablespoons crushed granola (modified)
- 1/4 teaspoon ground cinnamon

Instructions:

- In a bowl, combine cottage cheese, berries, and crushed granola.
- Sprinkle with cinnamon.

Tips:

- Choose lactose-free cottage cheese if you have lactose intolerance.
- Use different types of berries for variety.
- Top with a drizzle of low-fat maple syrup (once tolerated).

- 4. Egg Muffins with Vegetables and Cheese (approx. 150 calories, 8g protein, 8g carbohydrates, 8g fat):

Ingredients:

- 6 eggs
- 1/4 cup chopped vegetables (e.g., bell peppers, spinach, mushrooms)
- 1/4 cup shredded cheese (low-fat cheddar or mozzarella)
- Salt and pepper to taste
- Cooking spray

Instructions:

- Preheat oven to 375°F (190°C).
- Grease a muffin tin.
- Whisk together eggs, vegetables, and cheese in a bowl. Season with salt and pepper.
- Pour the mixture into the muffin tin cups.
- Bake for 15-20 minutes, or until eggs are set.

Tips:

- Use pre-chopped frozen vegetables for added convenience.
- Choose low-fiber vegetables like spinach or zucchini for easier digestion.
- Experiment

Smoothie Bowl with Tropical Fruits and Coconut Flakes

(approx. 300 calories, 15g protein, 40g carbohydrates, 10g fat):

Ingredients:

- 1/2 cup frozen mango
- 1/4 cup frozen pineapple
- 1/4 cup unsweetened coconut milk
- 1 tablespoon chia seeds

- 1 scoop protein powder (unflavored or vanilla) (optional)
- Toppings: Sliced banana, shredded coconut flakes, and a drizzle of honey (optional)

Instructions:

- Blend frozen fruits, coconut milk, chia seeds, and protein powder (if using) until smooth and creamy.
- Pour the smoothie into a bowl.
- Add your favorite toppings and enjoy.

Tips:

- Substitute frozen mango and pineapple with other frozen fruits like berries or papaya.
- Use unsweetened plant-based milk for a dairy-free option.
- Top with chopped nuts or seeds for added protein and healthy fats (once tolerated).
- 6. Overnight Oats with Berries and Nuts (approx. 250 calories, 10g protein, 40g carbohydrates, 5g fat):

Ingredients:

- 1/2 cup rolled oats
- 1/2 cup unsweetened almond milk
- 1/4 cup plain yogurt (unsweetened or low-sugar)
- 1/4 cup mixed berries
- 1 tablespoon chopped nuts (e.g., almonds, walnuts)
- 1/4 teaspoon ground cinnamon

Instructions:

- In a jar or container, combine rolled oats, almond milk, yogurt, berries, nuts, and cinnamon.
- Stir well, cover, and refrigerate overnight.
- Enjoy cold in the morning.

Tips:

- Choose different types of nuts and berries for variety.
- Substitute rolled oats with quick oats for a faster preparation.

- Add a teaspoon of chia seeds for additional fiber and nutrients.

Scrambled Tofu with Avocado and Tomatoes (approx. 200 calories, 15g protein, 15g carbohydrates, 10g fat):

Ingredients:

- 1/4 block firm tofu, crumbled
- 1/4 avocado, mashed
- 1/4 cup chopped tomatoes
- 1 tablespoon chopped onion
- 1/4 teaspoon turmeric powder
- Salt and pepper to taste
- Cooking spray

Instructions:

- Preheat a non-stick pan coated with cooking spray over medium heat.
- Saute onion until softened, about 1-2 minutes.
- Add crumbled tofu and turmeric powder. Cook for 2-3 minutes, stirring frequently.

- Stir in mashed avocado and chopped tomatoes.

- Season with salt and pepper to taste.

- Cook until warmed through.

Tips:

- Use pre-crumbled tofu for convenience.

- Add a splash of low-sodium vegetable broth for extra flavor.

- Substitute tomatoes with chopped spinach for a different vegetable option.

Chia Seed Pudding with Banana and Berries

(approx. 200 calories, 7g protein, 30g carbohydrates, 7g fat):

Ingredients:

- 1/4 cup chia seeds

- 1 cup unsweetened almond milk

- 1/4 cup mashed banana

- 1/4 cup mixed berries

- 1/4 teaspoon vanilla extract (optional)

Instructions:

- In a jar or container, combine chia seeds, almond milk, mashed banana, vanilla extract (if using), and stir well.
- Cover and refrigerate for at least 30 minutes, or overnight for a thicker consistency.
- Top with fresh berries before serving.

Tips:

- Use different types of fruits like mango or papaya for a different flavor.
- Sprinkle with a pinch of ground cinnamon for added flavor.
- Top with a dollop of low-fat yogurt for additional protein and creaminess (once tolerated).

Sweet Potato Toast with Eggs and Avocado

(approx. 250 calories, 12g protein, 25g carbohydrates, 10g fat):

Ingredients:

- 1 slice sweet potato, thinly sliced and toasted
- 2 eggs
- 1/4 avocado, sliced
- Salt and pepper to taste
- Cooking spray

Instructions:

- Preheat a non-stick pan coated with cooking spray over medium heat.
- Fry eggs to your desired doneness:
- For sunny-side up, cook until the whites are set and the yolks are runny.
- For over-easy, flip the eggs and cook for an additional 1-2 minutes until the yolks are slightly firm.
- For scrambled eggs, whisk the eggs in a bowl before adding them to the pan, then scramble until cooked through.
- Place the toasted sweet potato slice on a plate.
- Top with fried eggs and sliced avocado.

- Season with salt and pepper to taste.

Tips:

- Use a mandoline slicer for thin and even sweet potato slices.

- Toast the sweet potato slices in a toaster oven or air fryer for a healthier option.

- Substitute avocado with mashed banana or low-fat cream cheese (once tolerated) for a different topping.

- Drizzle with a teaspoon of hot sauce or sriracha for a kick (once tolerated).

- Sprinkle with chopped fresh herbs like chives or cilantro for added flavor.

- 10. Protein Pancakes with Berries and Yogurt (approx. 275 calories, 25g protein, 30g carbohydrates, 5g fat):

Ingredients:

- 1/2 cup cooked oatmeal

- 1 scoop protein powder (chocolate or vanilla)

- 1/4 cup unsweetened almond milk

- 1 egg

- 1/4 teaspoon baking powder

- 1/4 cup fresh berries

- 1/4 cup plain Greek yogurt (unsweetened or low-sugar)

Instructions:

- Blend all ingredients except berries and yogurt until smooth.

- Preheat a lightly greased non-stick pan over medium heat.

- Pour 1/4 cup of batter per pancake.

- Cook for 2-3 minutes per side, or until golden brown and cooked through.

- Serve pancakes topped with fresh berries and a dollop of Greek yogurt.

Tips:

- Use different protein powder flavors for variety.

- Add a pinch of stevia or a teaspoon of mashed banana for natural sweetness.

- Top with chopped nuts or seeds for added protein and healthy fats (once tolerated).

- 11. Veggie Frittata with Cheese (approx. 200 calories, 12g protein, 15g carbohydrates, 10g fat):

Ingredients:

- 2 eggs

- 1/4 cup chopped vegetables (e.g., bell peppers, spinach, mushrooms)

- 1/4 cup shredded cheese (low-fat cheddar or mozzarella)

- Salt and pepper to taste

- Cooking spray

Instructions:

- Preheat oven to 375°F (190°C).

- Heat a non-stick pan coated with cooking spray over medium heat.

- Add chopped vegetables and cook until softened, about 2-3 minutes.
- In a bowl, whisk together eggs, salt, and pepper.
- Pour the egg mixture into the pan with the vegetables.
- Sprinkle with cheese.
- Transfer the pan to the oven and bake for 10-15 minutes, or until the eggs are set and cheese is melted.

Tips:

- Choose low-fiber vegetables like spinach or zucchini for easier digestion.
- Use pre-chopped frozen vegetables for added convenience.
- Substitute cheese with chopped fresh herbs like parsley or chives for a different flavor profile.

Smoothie with Spinach, Banana, and Almond Butter (approx. 250 calories, 10g protein, 35g carbohydrates, 8g fat):

Ingredients:

- 1 cup unsweetened almond milk

- 1/2 banana, frozen

- 1 handful fresh spinach

- 1 tablespoon unsweetened almond butter

- 1/4 teaspoon ground cinnamon (optional)

Instructions:

- Blend all ingredients together until smooth and creamy.

- Enjoy chilled.

Tips:

- Substitute spinach with other leafy greens like kale or Swiss chard (once tolerated).

- Add a scoop of protein powder for an extra protein boost.

- Use different types of frozen fruit like berries or mango for variety.

- Egg Muffins with Ham and Vegetables (approx. 180 calories, 10g protein, 10g carbohydrates, 10g fat):

- 3. Egg Muffins with Ham and Vegetables (approx. 180 calories, 10g protein, 10g carbohydrates, 10g fat):

Ingredients:

- 6 eggs
- 1/4 cup chopped cooked ham
- 1/4 cup chopped vegetables (e.g., bell peppers, spinach, mushrooms)
- 1/4 cup shredded cheese (low-fat cheddar or mozzarella)
- Salt and pepper to taste
- Cooking spray

Instructions:

- Preheat oven to 375°F (190°C).

- Grease a muffin tin.

- In a large bowl, whisk together eggs, chopped ham, vegetables, and cheese. Season with salt and pepper to taste.

- Divide the egg mixture evenly among the muffin cups.

- Bake for 15-20 minutes, or until the eggs are set and the centers are no longer runny.

- Let cool slightly before removing from the muffin tin.

Tips:

- Use pre-cooked ham for convenience.

- Choose different types of vegetables for variety.

- Add a pinch of dried herbs like oregano or thyme for additional flavor.

- For a vegetarian option, omit the ham and add additional chopped vegetables.

- To make ahead of time, prepare the egg muffins and store them in an airtight container in the refrigerator for up to 3 days. Reheat in the microwave for a quick and easy breakfast.

Chapter 6:

Lunch and Dinner Recipes: Nutritious and Flavorful Options

Nourish your body with these flavorful and easy-to-follow recipes specifically designed for an ileostomy diet. This chapter offers a variety of options for lunch and dinner, featuring nutritious ingredients, clear instructions, and helpful tips.

Creamy Chicken and Vegetable Soup

(approx. 300 calories, 18g protein, 30g carbohydrates, 10g fat)

This comforting and satisfying soup provides essential nutrients and is gentle on the digestive system.

Ingredients:

- 1 tablespoon olive oil
- 1 onion (chopped)
- 1 carrot (chopped)
- 1 celery stalk (chopped)
- 4 cups chicken broth (low-sodium)
- 1 boneless, skinless chicken breast (cooked and shredded)
- 1/2 cup frozen peas
- 1/4 cup cooked rice
- 1/4 cup low-fat milk (or unsweetened plant-based milk)
- Salt and pepper to taste

Instructions:

- Heat olive oil in a large pot over medium heat.

- Add onion, carrot, and celery. Sauté for 5 minutes, or until softened.

- Pour in chicken broth and bring to a boil.

- Reduce heat, add shredded chicken, frozen peas, and cooked rice. Simmer for 10 minutes, or until peas are cooked through.

- Stir in milk and season with salt and pepper to taste.

- Serve hot.

Tips:

- Use leftover cooked chicken for added convenience.

- Choose low-fiber vegetables like zucchini or spinach for easier digestion.

- Substitute cooked quinoa or brown rice (if tolerated) for a different texture and additional fiber.

- Adjust the thickness of the soup by adding more or less broth or blending a portion for a smoother consistency.

- Recipe 2: Baked Salmon with Roasted Vegetables (approx. 350 calories, 25g protein, 20g carbohydrates, 15g fat)
- This baked salmon dish offers a protein and omega-3 fatty acid boost, paired with colorful roasted vegetables for a complete and flavorful meal.

Ingredients:

- 1 salmon fillet (6 oz)
- 1 tablespoon olive oil
- 1/2 teaspoon dried herbs (e.g., oregano, basil)
- Salt and pepper to taste
- 1 cup chopped vegetables (e.g., broccoli florets, cherry tomatoes, zucchini)

Instructions:

- Preheat oven to 400°F (200°C).
- Line a baking sheet with parchment paper.
- Season salmon fillet with olive oil, dried herbs, salt, and pepper.

- Toss chopped vegetables with a drizzle of olive oil and spread them on the baking sheet.

- Place the salmon fillet on top of the vegetables.

- Bake for 20-25 minutes, or until salmon is cooked through and vegetables are tender.

Tips:

- Choose other well-tolerated lean fish options like cod or tilapia.

- Marinate the salmon in lemon juice and herbs for added flavor (if tolerated).

- Experiment with different roasted vegetable combinations based on your preferences.

- Serve with cooked white rice or quinoa (if tolerated) for a complete meal.

Creamy Tomato Pasta Primavera

(approx. 350 calories, 20g protein, 40g carbohydrates, 10g fat)

This vibrant pasta dish features a creamy tomato sauce, lean protein, and a variety of low-fiber vegetables for a delightful and satisfying meal.

Ingredients:

- 1 tablespoon olive oil
- 1/2 onion (chopped)
- 1 clove garlic (minced)
- 1 (14.5 oz) can diced tomatoes (undrained)
- 1/4 cup low-fat milk (or unsweetened plant-based milk)
- 1/4 cup grated Parmesan cheese (optional)
- 1/4 cup cooked chicken breast (shredded) or other lean protein (e.g., shrimp, tofu)
- 1 cup cooked pasta (e.g., white penne, small shells)
- 1/2 cup chopped vegetables (e.g., bell peppers, spinach, mushrooms)
- Salt and pepper to taste

Instructions:

- Heat olive oil in a large pot over medium heat.

- Add onion and garlic, sauté for 2 minutes, or until softened.

- Stir in diced tomatoes and simmer for 5 minutes.

- Add milk and grated Parmesan cheese (if using). Season with salt and pepper to taste.

- In a separate pan, cook chosen protein (if using).

Chapter 7:

Snacking Smart: Healthy and Satisfying Choices

- Managing hunger and maintaining energy levels is crucial after ileostomy surgery. However, selecting the right snacks can be challenging. This chapter provides guidance on choosing healthy and satisfying options while following an ileostomy diet, along with delicious and easy-to-prepare snack recipes.

- *Importance of Healthy Snacking:*

- **Maintains energy levels:** Choosing nutrient-rich snacks throughout the day helps prevent dips in energy and keeps you feeling your best.

- **Supports healing**: Provides essential nutrients for healing and recovery.

- **Manages hunger**: Helps control hunger pangs and prevents overeating at mealtimes.

- **Hydration:** Choose options that contribute to your daily fluid intake.

Snacking Tips:

- **Plan ahead:** Prepare and portion snacks in advance to avoid unhealthy choices on the go.

- **Small and frequent:** Aim for smaller portions of snacks every 2-3 hours to avoid overwhelming your digestive system.

- **Variety is key:** Choose different snacks from various food groups to ensure you're getting a range of nutrients.

- **Focus on whole foods:** Opt for fresh fruits, vegetables, whole grains, and lean protein sources for optimal nutrition.

- **Read food labels:** Pay attention to ingredients, serving sizes, and sugar content, choosing low-fiber options when necessary.

- **Listen to your body:** Choose snacks that satisfy your hunger and cravings without causing discomfort.

Recipes

Homemade Trail Mix

(modified) (approx. 200 calories, 5g protein, 20g carbohydrates, 10g fat)

This customizable trail mix offers a satisfying blend of protein, healthy fats, and carbohydrates for sustained energy. Remember to modify this recipe based on your individual tolerances and preferences.

Ingredients:

- 1/4 cup dry roasted almonds (ground or finely chopped)
- 1/4 cup dried cranberries
- 1/4 cup pumpkin seeds
- 1/4 cup unsweetened shredded coconut flakes
- 1 tablespoon sunflower seeds

Instructions:

- Combine all ingredients in a bowl and mix well.
- Store in an airtight container for up to 5 days.

Tips:

- Substitute other nuts and seeds based on your tolerance and preferences (e.g., cashews, walnuts, sunflower seeds).
- Choose dried fruits with no added sugar for a healthier option.
- Add a small amount of dark chocolate chips (70% cacao or higher) for a touch of sweetness (once tolerated).

Yogurt with Berries and Chia Seeds

(approx. 150 calories, 8g protein, 20g carbohydrates, 3g fat)

This simple yet delicious snack combines creamy yogurt with the sweetness of berries and the added fiber and nutrients of chia seeds.

Ingredients:

- 1/2 cup plain yogurt (unsweetened or low-sugar)
- 1/4 cup fresh berries (e.g., blueberries, raspberries, strawberries)
- 1 tablespoon chia seeds

Instructions:

- Layer yogurt, berries, and chia seeds in a small bowl or container.
- Enjoy chilled.

Tips:

- Choose yogurt options labeled lactose-free if you have lactose intolerance.
- Substitute other chopped fruits like sliced banana or peaches for a different flavor combination.

- Sprinkle a touch of ground cinnamon or nutmeg for added flavor.

Rice Cakes with Nut Butter and Sliced Banana

(approx. 150 calories, 3g protein, 25g carbohydrates, 5g fat)

This classic snack provides a satisfying combination of complex carbohydrates from the rice cake, healthy fats from the nut butter, and natural sweetness from the banana.

Ingredients:

- 1 rice cake
- 2 tablespoons nut butter (smooth and no added sugar) (e.g., peanut butter, almond butter)
- 1/2 banana, sliced

Instructions:

- Spread nut butter evenly over the rice cake.
- Top with sliced banana.

Tips:

- Choose different types of rice cakes like brown rice or quinoa cakes for added nutrients (if tolerated).

- Substitute mashed avocado for nut butter for a different flavor and healthy fat option (once tolerated).

- Sprinkle a pinch of cinnamon for added flavor.

Part 4: Living Well with an Ileostomy

Chapter 8

Managing Common Digestive Issues: Tips and Solutions

Following ileostomy surgery, you might encounter new digestive challenges. This chapter equips you with information and strategies to manage common digestive issues like gas, bloating, diarrhea, and constipation, empowering you to take an active role in your well-being.

Understanding Common Digestive Issues:

- **Gas and bloating:** These can occur due to swallowing air while eating or drinking, consuming certain foods (e.g., beans, cruciferous vegetables), or bacterial fermentation in the digestive system.

- **Diarrhea:** Loose, frequent stools can happen due to various factors, including dietary changes, medications, or infections.

- **Constipation:** Difficulty passing stools can be caused by dehydration, lack of fiber in the diet, or medications.

Tips and Solutions:

Managing Gas and Bloating:

- **Eat slowly and chew thoroughly:** This allows for better digestion and minimizes air intake.

- **Identify and avoid trigger foods:** Keep a food diary to track your meals and any subsequent gas or bloating. Once you identify specific triggers, try to limit or avoid them.

- **Try herbal remedies:** Peppermint tea or ginger may help alleviate bloating and discomfort. (Consult your healthcare team before using any herbal remedies.)

- **Consider digestive enzymes:** Enzymes like lactase can help break down specific food components that might contribute to gas, but consult your healthcare team first.

Managing Diarrhea:

- **Stay hydrated:** Drink plenty of fluids to prevent dehydration, especially during diarrhea episodes.

- **BRAT diet:** This bland diet (bananas, rice, applesauce, and toast) is often recommended during short-term diarrhea episodes to help solidify stools.
- **Over-the-counter medications:** Consult your healthcare team about taking antidiarrheal medications for short-term relief.

Preventing Constipation:

➢ **Increase fiber intake:** Gradually introduce low-fiber fruits and vegetables (e.g., applesauce, well-cooked carrots) and low-fiber whole grains (e.g., white bread, cooked oats) into your diet as tolerated.

➢ **Hydrate adequately:** Drink plenty of water and other fluids throughout the day to soften stools.

➢ **Regular exercise:** Engaging in regular physical activity helps stimulate your digestive system.

Importance of Communication with your Healthcare Team:

➢ **Open communication:** Discuss any digestive concerns, changes in stool consistency or frequency, or any discomfort you experience with your healthcare team.

➤ **Do not hesitate to ask questions:** They are there to guide you and provide solutions to manage your individual needs.

➤ **Regular checkups**: Attend scheduled appointments and follow any recommendations or treatment plans your healthcare team suggests.

Additional Tips:

➤ **Manage stress:** Stress can exacerbate digestive issues. Practice relaxation techniques like deep breathing or meditation.

➤ **Maintain a healthy lifestyle:** Get enough sleep, engage in regular physical activity, and prioritize your well-being.

Join support groups: Connecting with others who understand your experience can be beneficial and offer emotional support.

By understanding these common digestive issues, adopting the suggested tips and strategies, and maintaining open communication with your healthcare team, you can effectively manage them and continue thriving with your ileostomy.

Chapter 9:

Maintaining Hydration: Strategies for Optimal Fluid Intake

Following ileostomy surgery, maintaining proper hydration becomes even more crucial. This chapter highlights the importance of water and electrolytes, explores various hydrating beverage options, and provides tips for monitoring your hydration levels throughout the day.

Importance of Water and Electrolytes:

> **Water:** It plays a vital role in digestion, nutrient absorption, and waste removal. Adequate water intake helps maintain the consistency of your stool and prevent constipation.

> **Electrolytes:** Minerals like sodium, potassium, and chloride are essential for maintaining fluid balance in your body. They also contribute to proper muscle function and nerve transmission.

Consequences of Dehydration:

Dehydration can lead to various complications, including:

> **Thicker stool:** This can increase the risk of constipation and straining, potentially leading to pouch prolapse or other complications.

> **Electrolyte imbalance:** This can cause fatigue, muscle cramps, dizziness, and even affect heart function.

> **Kidney stones:** Dehydration is a risk factor for developing kidney stones.

> **Choosing Healthy and Hydrating Beverages:**

> **Water:** Aim for plain water as your primary source of hydration.

> **Electrolyte-enhanced waters:** These can be helpful in replenishing electrolytes lost through your stoma output, but choose options with minimal added sugar.

> **Unsweetened herbal teas:** Offer additional flavor and variety while contributing to your fluid intake.

> **Diluted fruit juices:** Dilute 100% fruit juice with water in a 1:1 ratio to limit sugar intake.

➢ **Clear broths:** Low-sodium vegetable or chicken broths can provide additional hydration and electrolytes.

Tips for Monitoring Hydration Levels:

➢ **Monitor your urine color:** Pale yellow urine indicates adequate hydration, while darker urine suggests dehydration.

➢ **Track your fluid intake:** Keep a record of the amount of fluids you consume throughout the day. Aim for 8-10 glasses (2-2.5 liters) of water or other hydrating beverages. This is a general guideline, and your individual needs may vary based on factors like activity level and climate.

➢ **Observe your thirst:** While thirst is a natural cue, it can sometimes be unreliable after ileostomy surgery. Aim to stay ahead of thirst and drink fluids regularly throughout the day.

➢ **Monitor your weight:** Slight weight fluctuations are normal, but a sudden weight loss may indicate dehydration.

Additional Tips:

> **Carry a reusable water bottle:** Keep it with you throughout the day as a constant reminder to drink.

> **Set reminders:** Use your phone or a calendar app to set reminders to drink water at regular intervals.

> **Flavor your water:** Add slices of cucumber, lemon, or berries to your water for a subtle and refreshing taste.

> **Choose hydrating foods:** Include fruits and vegetables with high water content in your diet, such as watermelon, cucumber, and celery.

By prioritizing water and electrolyte intake, choosing healthy beverages, and monitoring your hydration levels, you can ensure your body receives the essential fluids it needs to function optimally and maintain overall well-being following ileostomy surgery. Remember, consulting your healthcare team for personalized hydration recommendations, especially regarding specific electrolyte needs and potential adjustments to your fluid intake, is crucial.

Chapter 10:

Long-Term Dietary Considerations and Support Resources

Living with an ileostomy is an ongoing journey, and maintaining a balanced diet is crucial for long-term health and well-being. This chapter discusses essential considerations for managing your diet over time, the importance of regular follow-up appointments, and resources available for support and guidance.

Maintaining a Balanced Diet Over Time:

✓ **Variety is key**: Continue incorporating a variety of food groups from different sources to ensure you're getting all the essential nutrients your body needs.

✓ **Gradual reintroduction**: Slowly reintroduce new foods under the guidance of your healthcare team, monitoring your tolerance and adjusting your diet as needed.

✓ **Balance fiber intake**: As your digestive system adapts, gradually increase low-fiber fruits, vegetables, and whole grains (if tolerated) to promote healthy digestion and prevent constipation.

✓ **Manage portion sizes**: Pay attention to portion sizes to avoid overeating and potential discomfort.

✓ **Stay hydrated**: Continue prioritizing adequate fluid intake to maintain proper hydration and prevent complications.

Importance of Regular Follow-up Appointments with your Healthcare Team:

✓ **Monitoring progress:** Regular checkups allow your healthcare team to monitor your overall health, stoma function, and nutritional status.

✓ **Adjusting dietary recommendations**: They can adjust your dietary recommendations based on your individual progress, tolerance, and any changes in your health.

✓ **Addressing concerns**: Discuss any ongoing digestive issues, concerns you might have, or questions about new foods you want to introduce.

✓ **Maintaining motivation and support**: Regular appointments provide a platform for continued support and motivation in managing your ileostomy and healthy lifestyle.

Finding Support Groups and Online Communities:

Connecting with others: Joining support groups or online communities can connect you with individuals who share similar experiences and offer emotional support, encouragement, and valuable insights.

✓ **Sharing experiences**: Sharing your experiences and learning from others can be empowering and provide valuable coping mechanisms for managing daily life with an ileostomy.

✓ **Accessing resources**: Support groups and online communities often offer access to educational resources, dietary tips, and recommendations for managing various aspects of living with an ileostomy.

Additional Tips:

- ✓ **Maintain a positive attitude**: A positive and optimistic outlook can significantly impact your overall well-being and ability to adapt to life with an ileostomy.
- ✓ **Celebrate your achievements**: Acknowledge your progress, no matter how small, and celebrate your journey.
- ✓ **Focus on living well**: Shift your focus from limitations to living a fulfilling and healthy life with your ileostomy.

Bonus

Ileostomy 7-Day Meal Plan with Recipes

Day 1:

- **Breakfast**: Scrambled Eggs with Vegetables and Toast (recipe in Chapter 5)

- **Lunch**: Tuna Salad Sandwich on White Bread with Lettuce and Tomato (recipe below)

- **Dinner:** Baked Chicken with Roasted Vegetables and Brown Rice (recipe below)

- **Snacks:** Sliced banana with almond butter, yogurt parfait with berries (modified recipe in Chapter 5)

Tuna Salad Sandwich:

Ingredients:

- 2 slices white bread

- 1 can (5 oz) tuna in water, drained

- 1 tablespoon light mayonnaise

- 1/4 cup chopped celery

- 1/4 teaspoon dried dill

- Salt and pepper to taste

Instructions:

- In a bowl, combine tuna, mayonnaise, celery, and dill. Season with salt and pepper to taste.
- Spread the tuna salad mixture on one slice of bread and top with the other slice.

Baked Chicken with Roasted Vegetables and Brown Rice:

Ingredients:

- 1 boneless, skinless chicken breast
- 1 tablespoon olive oil
- 1/2 teaspoon dried thyme
- Salt and pepper to taste
- 1 cup chopped vegetables (e.g., carrots, broccoli, potatoes)
- 1/2 cup cooked brown rice

Instructions:

- Preheat oven to 400°F (200°C).

- Season the chicken breast with olive oil, thyme, salt, and pepper.

- Place the chicken breast in a baking dish.

- Toss chopped vegetables with a drizzle of olive oil and spread around the chicken in the baking dish.

- Bake for 20-25 minutes, or until the chicken is cooked through and the vegetables are tender.

- Serve with cooked brown rice.

Day 2:

- **Breakfast:** Smoothie with Banana, Spinach, and Almond Milk (recipe below)

- **Lunch:** Chicken Caesar Salad with Grilled Chicken Breast (recipe below)

- **Dinner:** Salmon with Roasted Asparagus and Quinoa (recipe below)

- **Snacks:** Cottage cheese with berries and granola (modified recipe in Chapter 5), apple slices with peanut butter

Smoothie with Banana, Spinach, and Almond Milk:

Ingredients:

- 1/2 banana, frozen
- 1 handful fresh spinach
- 1 cup unsweetened almond milk
- 1/4 teaspoon ground cinnamon (optional)

Instructions:

- Blend all ingredients together until smooth and creamy.

- Enjoy chilled.

Chicken Caesar Salad with Grilled Chicken Breast:

Ingredients:

- 2 cups romaine lettuce, chopped

- 1 boneless, skinless chicken breast, grilled

- 1/4 cup shredded Parmesan cheese

- 2 tablespoons Caesar salad dressing (low-fat option)

- Croutons (optional, choose low-fiber options)

Instructions:

- Grill the chicken breast to your desired doneness.

- In a bowl, combine romaine lettuce, shredded Parmesan cheese, and Caesar salad dressing.

- Top with sliced grilled chicken and croutons (if using).

Salmon with Roasted Asparagus and Quinoa:

Ingredients:

- 1 salmon fillet

- 1 tablespoon olive oil

- Salt and pepper to taste

- 1 cup chopped asparagus

- 1/2 cup cooked quinoa

Instructions:

- Preheat oven to 400°F (200°C).

- Season the salmon fillet with olive oil, salt, and pepper.

- Place the salmon fillet on a baking sheet lined with parchment paper.

- Toss chopped asparagus with a drizzle of olive oil and spread around the salmon on the baking sheet.

- Bake for 15-20 minutes, or until the salmon is cooked through and the asparagus is tender-crisp.

- Serve with cooked quinoa.

Day 3

- **Breakfast:** Choose from Day 1 or Day 2 options, or explore other recipes in Chapter 5.

- **Lunch:** Choose from Day 1 or Day 2 options, or explore other protein and vegetable combinations.

- **Dinner:** Choose from Day 1 or Day 2 options, or explore other recipes suitable for an ileostomy diet.

- **Snacks:** Choose from Day 1 or Day 2 options, or explore other healthy and approved snack options.

Day 4:

- **Breakfast**: Protein Pancakes with Berries and Yogurt (recipe in Chapter 5)

- **Lunch**: Turkey and Vegetable Wrap with Whole Wheat Tortilla (recipe below)

- **Dinner**: Vegetarian Chili with Cornbread (recipe below)

- **Snacks**: Rice cakes with mashed avocado, sliced cucumber with hummus

Turkey and Vegetable Wrap with Whole Wheat Tortilla:

Ingredients:

- 1 whole wheat tortilla

- 3 ounces sliced turkey breast

- 1/4 cup chopped lettuce

- 1/4 cup chopped tomato

- 1 tablespoon light mayonnaise (optional)

- Salt and pepper to taste

Instructions:

- Spread a thin layer of mayonnaise (if using) onto the whole wheat tortilla.

- Layer the sliced turkey breast, lettuce, and tomato on the tortilla.

- Season with salt and pepper to taste.

- Roll up the tortilla tightly.

Vegetarian Chili with Cornbread:

Ingredients:

For the chili:

- 1 tablespoon olive oil

- 1 onion, chopped

- 1 green pepper, chopped

- 2 cloves garlic, minced

- 1 can (15 oz) diced tomatoes, undrained

- 1 can (15 oz) kidney beans, rinsed and drained

- 1 can (15 oz) black beans, rinsed and drained

- 1 cup vegetable broth

- 1/2 teaspoon chili powder

- 1/4 teaspoon cumin

- Salt and pepper to taste

For the cornbread:

- 1/2 cup self-rising cornmeal

- 1/4 cup all-purpose flour

- 1/4 cup sugar

- 1/2 teaspoon baking powder

- 1/4 teaspoon salt

- 1 egg

- 1/3 cup milk

- 1 tablespoon melted butter

Instructions:

- For the chili: Heat olive oil in a large pot over medium heat.

- Add onion and green pepper, and cook until softened, about 5 minutes.

- Add garlic and cook for an additional minute.

- Stir in diced tomatoes, kidney beans, black beans, vegetable broth, chili powder, and cumin.

- Bring to a boil, then reduce heat and simmer for 20-25 minutes, or until slightly thickened.

- Season with salt and pepper to taste.

For the cornbread:

- Preheat oven to 400°F (200°C). Grease a small baking dish.

- In a bowl, whisk together cornmeal, flour, sugar, baking powder, and salt.

- In another bowl, whisk together egg and milk.

- Add the wet ingredients to the dry ingredients and stir until just combined.

- Fold in melted butter.

- Pour the batter into the prepared baking dish.

- Bake for 15-20 minutes, or until a toothpick inserted into the center comes out clean.

Day 5:

- **Breakfast:** Overnight Oats with Berries and Nuts (recipe in Chapter 5)

- **Lunch:** Chicken Noodle Soup with Whole Wheat Bread (recipe below)

- **Dinner:** Baked Cod with Roasted Sweet Potatoes and Green Beans (recipe below)
- **Snacks:** Sliced apple with almond butter, yogurt with granola and berries (modified recipe in Chapter 5)

Chicken Noodle Soup with Whole Wheat Bread:

Ingredients:

- 4 cups chicken broth
- 1 boneless, skinless chicken breast, cooked and shredded
- 1/2 cup chopped carrots
- 1/2 cup chopped celery
- 1/4 cup chopped onion
- 1/4 cup dried egg noodles
- Salt and pepper to taste
- 1 slice whole wheat bread

Instructions:

- In a large pot, bring chicken broth to a boil.

- Add carrots, celery, and onion.

- Reduce heat and simmer for 10 minutes, or until vegetables are tender.

- Add shredded chicken and dried egg noodles.

- Cook for an additional 5 minutes, or until the noodles are cooked through.

- Season with salt and pepper to taste.

- Serve with a slice of whole wheat bread.

Baked Cod with Roasted Sweet Potatoes and Green Beans:

Ingredients:

- 1 cod fillet

- 1 tablespoon olive oil

- Salt and pepper to taste

- 1 medium sweet potato, peeled and diced

- 1 cup green beans, trimmed

Instructions:

- Preheat oven to 400°F (20

- Toss diced sweet potato and green beans with olive oil, salt, and pepper.

- Spread the vegetables on a baking sheet.

- Place the cod fillet on top of the vegetables.

- Bake for 20-25 minutes, or until the cod is cooked through and the vegetables are tender-crisp.

Day 6:

- **Breakfast:** Scrambled Eggs with Spinach and Cheese (recipe below)
- **Lunch:** Lentil Soup with Whole Wheat Roll (recipe below)
- **Dinner:** Grilled Chicken Breast with Brown Rice and Steamed Broccoli (recipe below)
- **Snacks:** Pear slices with string cheese, carrot sticks with hummus

Scrambled Eggs with Spinach and Cheese:

Ingredients:

- 2 eggs
- 1 tablespoon olive oil
- 1/4 cup chopped spinach
- 1/4 cup shredded cheese (low-fat cheddar or mozzarella)
- Salt and pepper to taste

Instructions:

- Heat olive oil in a non-stick pan over medium heat.

- Add chopped spinach and cook until wilted, about 2 minutes.

- Push the spinach to one side of the pan.

- In the empty space, whisk together the eggs.

- Scramble the eggs until desired doneness, then combine with the spinach.

- Sprinkle with shredded cheese and cook for an additional minute, or until the cheese is melted.

- Season with salt and pepper to taste.

Lentil Soup with Whole Wheat Roll:

Ingredients:

For the soup:

- 1 tablespoon olive oil

- 1 onion, chopped

- 1 carrot, chopped

- 1 celery stalk, chopped

- 2 cloves garlic, minced

- 1 can (15 oz) diced tomatoes, undrained

- 1 cup vegetable broth

- 1 cup green lentils, rinsed
- 1/2 teaspoon dried thyme
- Salt and pepper to taste

For the whole wheat roll:

- 1 small whole wheat roll

Instructions:

For the soup:

- Heat olive oil in a large pot over medium heat.
- Add onion, carrot, and celery, and cook until softened, about 5 minutes.
- Add garlic and cook for an additional minute.
- Stir in diced tomatoes, vegetable broth, lentils, and thyme.
- Bring to a boil, then reduce heat and simmer for 30-35 minutes, or until lentils are tender.
- Season with salt and pepper to taste.

For the whole wheat roll:

Warm the whole wheat roll according to package instructions.

Grilled Chicken Breast with Brown Rice and Steamed Broccoli:

Ingredients:

- 1 boneless, skinless chicken breast
- 1 tablespoon olive oil
- Salt and pepper to taste
- 1/2 cup cooked brown rice
- 1 cup steamed broccoli florets

Instructions:

- Preheat grill to medium heat.
- Brush the chicken breast with olive oil and season with salt and pepper.
- Grill the chicken breast for 5-7 minutes per side, or until cooked through.
- Serve with cooked brown rice and steamed broccoli florets.

Day 7:

- **Breakfast:** Smoothie with Banana, Yogurt, and Berries (recipe below)
- **Lunch**: Chicken Salad Sandwich on Whole Wheat Bread with Lettuce and Tomato (recipe below)
- **Dinner**: Salmon with Roasted Brussels Sprouts and Quinoa (recipe below)
- **Snacks:** Cottage cheese with pineapple chunks, sliced cucumber with Greek yogurt dip

Smoothie with Banana, Yogurt, and Berries:

Ingredients:

- 1/2 banana, frozen
- 1/2 cup plain Greek yogurt
- 1/4 cup mixed berries
- 1/4 cup unsweetened almond milk
- 1/4 teaspoon ground cinnamon (optional)

Instructions:

- Blend all ingredients together until smooth and creamy.

- Enjoy chilled.

Chicken Salad Sandwich on Whole Wheat Bread with Lettuce and Tomato:

Ingredients:

- 2 slices whole wheat bread

- 3 ounces cooked and shredded chicken breast

- 1 tablespoon light mayonnaise

- 1/4 cup chopped celery

- 1/4 cup chopped lettuce

- 1/4 cup sliced tomato

- Salt and pepper to taste

Instructions:

- In a bowl, combine shredded chicken, mayonnaise, and celery. Season with salt and pepper to taste.

- Spread the chicken salad mixture on one slice of whole wheat bread.

- Top with lettuce and tomato slices.

- Place the other slice of bread on top.

Salmon with Roasted Brussels Sprouts and Quinoa:

Ingredients:

- 1 salmon fillet
- 1 tablespoon olive oil
- Salt and pepper to taste
- 1 cup Brussels sprouts, trimmed and halved
- 1/2 cup cooked quinoa

Instructions:

- Preheat oven to 400°F (200°C).
- Toss Brussels sprouts with olive oil, salt, and pepper.
- Spread the Brussels sprouts on a baking sheet.
- Place the salmon fillet on top of the Brussels sprouts.
- Bake for 15-20 minutes, or until the salmon is cooked through and the Brussels sprouts are tender-crisp.
- Serve with cooked quinoa.

Remember:

This is just a sample plan, and you may need to adjust it based on your individual needs and preferences.

Always consult with your healthcare team to create a personalized plan that meets your specific requirements.

- Continue to monitor your tolerance to different foods and adjust your diet accordingly.

Additional Tips:

- Explore different recipes that are suitable for an ileostomy diet.
- Experiment with various herbs and spices to add flavor to your meals.
- Consider incorporating low-fiber fruits and vegetables into your diet, such as bananas, applesauce, carrots, and green beans.
- Listen to your body and avoid foods that trigger negative symptoms.

- By following these tips and incorporating a variety of healthy options, you can manage your ileostomy effectively and maintain a balanced and nutritious diet.

Conclusion:

Embracing a New Chapter with Delicious Options

Living with an ileostomy may require dietary adjustments, but it doesn't have to limit your culinary experiences. This cookbook serves as a guide to empower you on your journey, equipping you with delicious and nutritious recipes specifically designed for an ileostomy diet.

Throughout this book, we explored a variety of meal options, from easy-to-prepare breakfasts to satisfying lunches and dinners, along with healthy snacking ideas. Remember, these recipes are just a starting point, and a world of delicious possibilities awaits your exploration.

As you embark on this new chapter, embrace the opportunity to discover new flavors and culinary creations. Experiment with different ingredients, personalize recipes based on your preferences, and most importantly, enjoy the journey of creating delicious and nutritious meals that fuel your body and enrich your life.

www.ingramcontent.com/pod-product-compliance
Lightning Source LLC
Chambersburg PA
CBHW070758260726
48660CB00005B/1682